VITAL SIGNS LOG BOOK

INFORMATION

Name	
Phone No.	
Fax No.	Email
Address	
Other Contact	

IMPORTANT DOCTOR, CLINIC, HOSPITAL CONTACTS

Name	Phone - Fax - Email

Copyright © All Rights Reserved by Logbooks Simon

Date:		Wt. (am);	(pm);
Name:			
	Morning	Mid-Day	Night
Blood Pressure	/	/	/
Heart Rate			
Oxygen Level			
Blood Sugar			
Temperature			

Notes _____
_____
_____
_____

Date:		Wt. (am);	(pm);
Name:			
	Morning	Mid-Day	Night
Blood Pressure	/	/	/
Heart Rate			
Oxygen Level			
Blood Sugar			
Temperature			

Notes _____
_____
_____
_____

Date:		Wt. (am);	(pm);
Name:			
	Morning	Mid-Day	Night
Blood Pressure	/	/	/
Heart Rate			
Oxygen Level			
Blood Sugar			
Temperature			

Notes _____
_____
_____
_____

Date:		Wt. (am);	(pm);
Name:			
	Morning	Mid-Day	Night
Blood Pressure	/	/	/
Heart Rate			
Oxygen Level			
Blood Sugar			
Temperature			

Notes _____
_____
_____
_____

Date:		Wt. (am);	(pm);
Name:			
	Morning	Mid-Day	Night
Blood Pressure	/	/	/
Heart Rate			
Oxygen Level			
Blood Sugar			
Temperature			

Notes _____
_____
_____
_____

Date:		Wt. (am);	(pm);
Name:			
	Morning	Mid-Day	Night
Blood Pressure	/	/	/
Heart Rate			
Oxygen Level			
Blood Sugar			
Temperature			

Notes _____
_____
_____
_____

Date:		Wt. (am);	(pm);
Name:			
	Morning	Mid-Day	Night
Blood Pressure	/	/	/
Heart Rate			
Oxygen Level			
Blood Sugar			
Temperature			

Notes _____
_____
_____
_____

Date:		Wt. (am);	(pm);
Name:			
	Morning	Mid-Day	Night
Blood Pressure	/	/	/
Heart Rate			
Oxygen Level			
Blood Sugar			
Temperature			

Notes _____
_____
_____
_____

Date:		Wt. (am);	(pm);
Name:			
	Morning	Mid-Day	Night
Blood Pressure	/	/	/
Heart Rate			
Oxygen Level			
Blood Sugar			
Temperature			

Notes _____
_____
_____

Date:		Wt. (am);	(pm);
Name:			
	Morning	Mid-Day	Night
Blood Pressure	/	/	/
Heart Rate			
Oxygen Level			
Blood Sugar			
Temperature			

Notes _____
_____
_____

Date: Wt. (am);   (pm);

Name:

	Morning	Mid-Day	Night
Blood Pressure	/	/	/
Heart Rate			
Oxygen Level			
Blood Sugar			
Temperature			

Notes _____
_____
_____
_____

Date: Wt. (am);   (pm);

Name:

	Morning	Mid-Day	Night
Blood Pressure	/	/	/
Heart Rate			
Oxygen Level			
Blood Sugar			
Temperature			

Notes _____
_____
_____
_____

Date:	Wt. (am);		(pm);
Name:			
	Morning	Mid-Day	Night
Blood Pressure	/	/	/
Heart Rate			
Oxygen Level			
Blood Sugar			
Temperature			

Notes _____

_____

_____

_____

Date:	Wt. (am);		(pm);
Name:			
	Morning	Mid-Day	Night
Blood Pressure	/	/	/
Heart Rate			
Oxygen Level			
Blood Sugar			
Temperature			

Notes _____

_____

_____

_____

Date:		Wt. (am);		(pm);
Name:				
	Morning	Mid-Day		Night
Blood Pressure	/	/		/
Heart Rate				
Oxygen Level				
Blood Sugar				
Temperature				

Notes _____
_____
_____
_____

Date:		Wt. (am);		(pm);
Name:				
	Morning	Mid-Day		Night
Blood Pressure	/	/		/
Heart Rate				
Oxygen Level				
Blood Sugar				
Temperature				

Notes _____
_____
_____
_____

Date:		Wt. (am);	(pm);
Name:			
	Morning	Mid-Day	Night
Blood Pressure	/	/	/
Heart Rate			
Oxygen Level			
Blood Sugar			
Temperature			

Notes _____

_____

_____

_____

Date:		Wt. (am);	(pm);
Name:			
	Morning	Mid-Day	Night
Blood Pressure	/	/	/
Heart Rate			
Oxygen Level			
Blood Sugar			
Temperature			

Notes _____

_____

_____

_____

Date:		Wt. (am);	(pm);
Name:			
	Morning	Mid-Day	Night
Blood Pressure	/	/	/
Heart Rate			
Oxygen Level			
Blood Sugar			
Temperature			

Notes _____
_____
_____
_____

Date:		Wt. (am);	(pm);
Name:			
	Morning	Mid-Day	Night
Blood Pressure	/	/	/
Heart Rate			
Oxygen Level			
Blood Sugar			
Temperature			

Notes _____
_____
_____
_____

Date:		Wt. (am);	(pm);
Name:			
	Morning	Mid-Day	Night
Blood Pressure	/	/	/
Heart Rate			
Oxygen Level			
Blood Sugar			
Temperature			

Notes _____

_____

_____

_____

Date:		Wt. (am);	(pm);
Name:			
	Morning	Mid-Day	Night
Blood Pressure	/	/	/
Heart Rate			
Oxygen Level			
Blood Sugar			
Temperature			

Notes _____

_____

_____

_____

Date: _____ Wt. (am); _____ (pm); _____

Name: _____

	Morning	Mid-Day	Night
Blood Pressure	/	/	/
Heart Rate			
Oxygen Level			
Blood Sugar			
Temperature			

Notes _____
_____
_____
_____

Date: _____ Wt. (am); _____ (pm); _____

Name: _____

	Morning	Mid-Day	Night
Blood Pressure	/	/	/
Heart Rate			
Oxygen Level			
Blood Sugar			
Temperature			

Notes _____
_____
_____
_____

Date:		Wt. (am);	(pm);
Name:			
	Morning	Mid-Day	Night
Blood Pressure	/	/	/
Heart Rate			
Oxygen Level			
Blood Sugar			
Temperature			

Notes _____
_____
_____
_____

Date:		Wt. (am);	(pm);
Name:			
	Morning	Mid-Day	Night
Blood Pressure	/	/	/
Heart Rate			
Oxygen Level			
Blood Sugar			
Temperature			

Notes _____
_____
_____
_____

Date:		Wt. (am);	(pm);
Name:			
	Morning	Mid-Day	Night
Blood Pressure	/	/	/
Heart Rate			
Oxygen Level			
Blood Sugar			
Temperature			

Notes _____

_____

_____

_____

Date:		Wt. (am);	(pm);
Name:			
	Morning	Mid-Day	Night
Blood Pressure	/	/	/
Heart Rate			
Oxygen Level			
Blood Sugar			
Temperature			

Notes _____

_____

_____

_____

Date:		Wt. (am);	(pm);
Name:			
	Morning	Mid-Day	Night
Blood Pressure	/	/	/
Heart Rate			
Oxygen Level			
Blood Sugar			
Temperature			

Notes _____
_____
_____
_____

Date:		Wt. (am);	(pm);
Name:			
	Morning	Mid-Day	Night
Blood Pressure	/	/	/
Heart Rate			
Oxygen Level			
Blood Sugar			
Temperature			

Notes _____
_____
_____
_____

Date: Wt. (am);   (pm);

Name:

	Morning	Mid-Day	Night
Blood Pressure	/	/	/
Heart Rate			
Oxygen Level			
Blood Sugar			
Temperature			

Notes _____
_____
_____

Date: Wt. (am);   (pm);

Name:

	Morning	Mid-Day	Night
Blood Pressure	/	/	/
Heart Rate			
Oxygen Level			
Blood Sugar			
Temperature			

Notes _____
_____
_____

Date:		Wt. (am);	(pm);
Name:			
	Morning	Mid-Day	Night
Blood Pressure	/	/	/
Heart Rate			
Oxygen Level			
Blood Sugar			
Temperature			

Notes _____

_____

_____

_____

Date:		Wt. (am);	(pm);
Name:			
	Morning	Mid-Day	Night
Blood Pressure	/	/	/
Heart Rate			
Oxygen Level			
Blood Sugar			
Temperature			

Notes _____

_____

_____

_____

Date:		Wt. (am);		(pm);	
Name:					
	Morning		Mid-Day		Night
Blood Pressure	/		/		/
Heart Rate					
Oxygen Level					
Blood Sugar					
Temperature					

Notes _____

_____

_____

_____

Date:		Wt. (am);		(pm);	
Name:					
	Morning		Mid-Day		Night
Blood Pressure	/		/		/
Heart Rate					
Oxygen Level					
Blood Sugar					
Temperature					

Notes _____

_____

_____

_____

Date:		Wt. (am);	(pm);
Name:			
	Morning	Mid-Day	Night
Blood Pressure	/	/	/
Heart Rate			
Oxygen Level			
Blood Sugar			
Temperature			

Notes _____
_____
_____
_____

Date:		Wt. (am);	(pm);
Name:			
	Morning	Mid-Day	Night
Blood Pressure	/	/	/
Heart Rate			
Oxygen Level			
Blood Sugar			
Temperature			

Notes _____
_____
_____
_____

Date:		Wt. (am);	(pm);
Name:			
	Morning	Mid-Day	Night
Blood Pressure	/	/	/
Heart Rate			
Oxygen Level			
Blood Sugar			
Temperature			

Notes _____

_____

_____

_____

Date:		Wt. (am);	(pm);
Name:			
	Morning	Mid-Day	Night
Blood Pressure	/	/	/
Heart Rate			
Oxygen Level			
Blood Sugar			
Temperature			

Notes _____

_____

_____

_____

Date:		Wt. (am);	(pm);
Name:			
	Morning	Mid-Day	Night
Blood Pressure	/	/	/
Heart Rate			
Oxygen Level			
Blood Sugar			
Temperature			

Notes _____
_____
_____
_____

Date:		Wt. (am);	(pm);
Name:			
	Morning	Mid-Day	Night
Blood Pressure	/	/	/
Heart Rate			
Oxygen Level			
Blood Sugar			
Temperature			

Notes _____
_____
_____
_____

Date:		Wt. (am);	(pm);
Name:			
	Morning	Mid-Day	Night
Blood Pressure	/	/	/
Heart Rate			
Oxygen Level			
Blood Sugar			
Temperature			

Notes _____
_____
_____
_____

Date:		Wt. (am);	(pm);
Name:			
	Morning	Mid-Day	Night
Blood Pressure	/	/	/
Heart Rate			
Oxygen Level			
Blood Sugar			
Temperature			

Notes _____
_____
_____
_____

Date:		Wt. (am);	(pm);
Name:			
	Morning	Mid-Day	Night
Blood Pressure	/	/	/
Heart Rate			
Oxygen Level			
Blood Sugar			
Temperature			

Notes _____
_____
_____
_____

Date:		Wt. (am);	(pm);
Name:			
	Morning	Mid-Day	Night
Blood Pressure	/	/	/
Heart Rate			
Oxygen Level			
Blood Sugar			
Temperature			

Notes _____
_____
_____
_____

Date:		Wt. (am);		(pm);
Name:				
	Morning	Mid-Day		Night
Blood Pressure	/	/		/
Heart Rate				
Oxygen Level				
Blood Sugar				
Temperature				

Notes _____

_____

_____

_____

Date:		Wt. (am);		(pm);
Name:				
	Morning	Mid-Day		Night
Blood Pressure	/	/		/
Heart Rate				
Oxygen Level				
Blood Sugar				
Temperature				

Notes _____

_____

_____

_____

Date:		Wt. (am);	(pm);
Name:			
	Morning	Mid-Day	Night
Blood Pressure	/	/	/
Heart Rate			
Oxygen Level			
Blood Sugar			
Temperature			

Notes _____

_____

_____

_____

Date:		Wt. (am);	(pm);
Name:			
	Morning	Mid-Day	Night
Blood Pressure	/	/	/
Heart Rate			
Oxygen Level			
Blood Sugar			
Temperature			

Notes _____

_____

_____

_____

Date: Wt. (am); (pm);

Name:

	Morning	Mid-Day	Night
Blood Pressure	/	/	/
Heart Rate			
Oxygen Level			
Blood Sugar			
Temperature			

Notes _____
_____
_____
_____

Date: Wt. (am); (pm);

Name:

	Morning	Mid-Day	Night
Blood Pressure	/	/	/
Heart Rate			
Oxygen Level			
Blood Sugar			
Temperature			

Notes _____
_____
_____
_____

Date:		Wt. (am);	(pm);
Name:			
	Morning	Mid-Day	Night
Blood Pressure	/	/	/
Heart Rate			
Oxygen Level			
Blood Sugar			
Temperature			

Notes _____

_____

_____

_____

Date:		Wt. (am);	(pm);
Name:			
	Morning	Mid-Day	Night
Blood Pressure	/	/	/
Heart Rate			
Oxygen Level			
Blood Sugar			
Temperature			

Notes _____

_____

_____

_____

Date:		Wt. (am);	(pm);
Name:			
	Morning	Mid-Day	Night
Blood Pressure	/	/	/
Heart Rate			
Oxygen Level			
Blood Sugar			
Temperature			

Notes _____
_____
_____
_____

Date:		Wt. (am);	(pm);
Name:			
	Morning	Mid-Day	Night
Blood Pressure	/	/	/
Heart Rate			
Oxygen Level			
Blood Sugar			
Temperature			

Notes _____
_____
_____
_____

Date:	Wt. (am);	(pm);	
Name:			
	Morning	Mid-Day	Night
Blood Pressure	/	/	/
Heart Rate			
Oxygen Level			
Blood Sugar			
Temperature			

Notes _____
_____
_____
_____

Date:	Wt. (am);	(pm);	
Name:			
	Morning	Mid-Day	Night
Blood Pressure	/	/	/
Heart Rate			
Oxygen Level			
Blood Sugar			
Temperature			

Notes _____
_____
_____
_____

Date: _____ Wt. (am); _____ (pm); _____
Name: _____

	Morning	Mid-Day	Night
Blood Pressure	/	/	/
Heart Rate			
Oxygen Level			
Blood Sugar			
Temperature			

Notes _____

_____

_____

Date: _____ Wt. (am); _____ (pm); _____
Name: _____

	Morning	Mid-Day	Night
Blood Pressure	/	/	/
Heart Rate			
Oxygen Level			
Blood Sugar			
Temperature			

Notes _____

_____

_____

Date:		Wt. (am);	(pm);
Name:			
	Morning	Mid-Day	Night
Blood Pressure	/	/	/
Heart Rate			
Oxygen Level			
Blood Sugar			
Temperature			

Notes _____

_____

_____

_____

Date:		Wt. (am);	(pm);
Name:			
	Morning	Mid-Day	Night
Blood Pressure	/	/	/
Heart Rate			
Oxygen Level			
Blood Sugar			
Temperature			

Notes _____

_____

_____

_____

Date:		Wt. (am);	(pm);
Name:			
	Morning	Mid-Day	Night
Blood Pressure	/	/	/
Heart Rate			
Oxygen Level			
Blood Sugar			
Temperature			

Notes _____

_____

_____

_____

Date:		Wt. (am);	(pm);
Name:			
	Morning	Mid-Day	Night
Blood Pressure	/	/	/
Heart Rate			
Oxygen Level			
Blood Sugar			
Temperature			

Notes _____

_____

_____

_____

Date:		Wt. (am);	(pm);
Name:			
	Morning	Mid-Day	Night
Blood Pressure	/	/	/
Heart Rate			
Oxygen Level			
Blood Sugar			
Temperature			

Notes _____

_____

_____

_____

Date:		Wt. (am);	(pm);
Name:			
	Morning	Mid-Day	Night
Blood Pressure	/	/	/
Heart Rate			
Oxygen Level			
Blood Sugar			
Temperature			

Notes _____

_____

_____

_____

Date:		Wt. (am);	(pm);
Name:			
	Morning	Mid-Day	Night
Blood Pressure	/	/	/
Heart Rate			
Oxygen Level			
Blood Sugar			
Temperature			

Notes _____
_____
_____
_____

Date:		Wt. (am);	(pm);
Name:			
	Morning	Mid-Day	Night
Blood Pressure	/	/	/
Heart Rate			
Oxygen Level			
Blood Sugar			
Temperature			

Notes _____
_____
_____
_____

Date:		Wt. (am);	(pm);
Name:			
	Morning	Mid-Day	Night
Blood Pressure	/	/	/
Heart Rate			
Oxygen Level			
Blood Sugar			
Temperature			

Notes _____

_____

_____

_____

Date:		Wt. (am);	(pm);
Name:			
	Morning	Mid-Day	Night
Blood Pressure	/	/	/
Heart Rate			
Oxygen Level			
Blood Sugar			
Temperature			

Notes _____

_____

_____

_____

Date: Wt. (am);   (pm);

Name:

	Morning	Mid-Day	Night
Blood Pressure	/	/	/
Heart Rate			
Oxygen Level			
Blood Sugar			
Temperature			

Notes _____
_____
_____
_____

Date: Wt. (am);   (pm);

Name:

	Morning	Mid-Day	Night
Blood Pressure	/	/	/
Heart Rate			
Oxygen Level			
Blood Sugar			
Temperature			

Notes _____
_____
_____
_____

Date:		Wt. (am);	(pm);
Name:			
	Morning	Mid-Day	Night
Blood Pressure	/	/	/
Heart Rate			
Oxygen Level			
Blood Sugar			
Temperature			

Notes _____

_____

_____

_____

Date:		Wt. (am);	(pm);
Name:			
	Morning	Mid-Day	Night
Blood Pressure	/	/	/
Heart Rate			
Oxygen Level			
Blood Sugar			
Temperature			

Notes _____

_____

_____

_____

Date:		Wt. (am);		(pm);
Name:				
	Morning	Mid-Day		Night
Blood Pressure	/	/		/
Heart Rate				
Oxygen Level				
Blood Sugar				
Temperature				

Notes _____
_____
_____
_____

Date:		Wt. (am);		(pm);
Name:				
	Morning	Mid-Day		Night
Blood Pressure	/	/		/
Heart Rate				
Oxygen Level				
Blood Sugar				
Temperature				

Notes _____
_____
_____
_____

Date:		Wt. (am);	(pm);
Name:			

	Morning	Mid-Day	Night
Blood Pressure	/	/	/
Heart Rate			
Oxygen Level			
Blood Sugar			
Temperature			

Notes _____

_____

_____

_____

Date:		Wt. (am);	(pm);
Name:			

	Morning	Mid-Day	Night
Blood Pressure	/	/	/
Heart Rate			
Oxygen Level			
Blood Sugar			
Temperature			

Notes _____

_____

_____

_____

Date:		Wt. (am);	(pm);
Name:			
	Morning	Mid-Day	Night
Blood Pressure	/	/	/
Heart Rate			
Oxygen Level			
Blood Sugar			
Temperature			

Notes _____
_____
_____
_____

Date:		Wt. (am);	(pm);
Name:			
	Morning	Mid-Day	Night
Blood Pressure	/	/	/
Heart Rate			
Oxygen Level			
Blood Sugar			
Temperature			

Notes _____
_____
_____
_____

Date: Wt. (am);   (pm);

Name:

	Morning	Mid-Day	Night
Blood Pressure	/	/	/
Heart Rate			
Oxygen Level			
Blood Sugar			
Temperature			

Notes _____

_____

_____

_____

Date: Wt. (am);   (pm);

Name:

	Morning	Mid-Day	Night
Blood Pressure	/	/	/
Heart Rate			
Oxygen Level			
Blood Sugar			
Temperature			

Notes _____

_____

_____

_____

Date: _____ Wt. (am); _____ (pm); _____

Name: _____

	Morning	Mid-Day	Night
Blood Pressure	/	/	/
Heart Rate			
Oxygen Level			
Blood Sugar			
Temperature			

Notes _____
_____
_____
_____

Date: _____ Wt. (am); _____ (pm); _____

Name: _____

	Morning	Mid-Day	Night
Blood Pressure	/	/	/
Heart Rate			
Oxygen Level			
Blood Sugar			
Temperature			

Notes _____
_____
_____
_____

Date:	Wt. (am);		(pm);
Name:			

	Morning	Mid-Day	Night
Blood Pressure	/	/	/
Heart Rate			
Oxygen Level			
Blood Sugar			
Temperature			

Notes _____

_____

_____

_____

Date:	Wt. (am);		(pm);
Name:			

	Morning	Mid-Day	Night
Blood Pressure	/	/	/
Heart Rate			
Oxygen Level			
Blood Sugar			
Temperature			

Notes _____

_____

_____

_____

Date: _____ Wt. (am); _____ (pm); _____

Name: _____

	Morning	Mid-Day	Night
Blood Pressure	/	/	/
Heart Rate			
Oxygen Level			
Blood Sugar			
Temperature			

Notes _____
_____
_____

Date: _____ Wt. (am); _____ (pm); _____

Name: _____

	Morning	Mid-Day	Night
Blood Pressure	/	/	/
Heart Rate			
Oxygen Level			
Blood Sugar			
Temperature			

Notes _____
_____
_____

Date:		Wt. (am);	(pm);
Name:			
	Morning	Mid-Day	Night
Blood Pressure	/	/	/
Heart Rate			
Oxygen Level			
Blood Sugar			
Temperature			

Notes _____

_____

_____

Date:		Wt. (am);	(pm);
Name:			
	Morning	Mid-Day	Night
Blood Pressure	/	/	/
Heart Rate			
Oxygen Level			
Blood Sugar			
Temperature			

Notes _____

_____

_____

Date:		Wt. (am);	(pm);
Name:			
	Morning	Mid-Day	Night
Blood Pressure	/	/	/
Heart Rate			
Oxygen Level			
Blood Sugar			
Temperature			

Notes _____

_____

_____

Date:		Wt. (am);	(pm);
Name:			
	Morning	Mid-Day	Night
Blood Pressure	/	/	/
Heart Rate			
Oxygen Level			
Blood Sugar			
Temperature			

Notes _____

_____

_____

Date:		Wt. (am);	(pm);
Name:			
	Morning	Mid-Day	Night
Blood Pressure	/	/	/
Heart Rate			
Oxygen Level			
Blood Sugar			
Temperature			

Notes _____
_____
_____
_____

Date:		Wt. (am);	(pm);
Name:			
	Morning	Mid-Day	Night
Blood Pressure	/	/	/
Heart Rate			
Oxygen Level			
Blood Sugar			
Temperature			

Notes _____
_____
_____
_____

Date: _____ Wt. (am); _____ (pm); _____

Name: _____

	Morning	Mid-Day	Night
Blood Pressure	/	/	/
Heart Rate			
Oxygen Level			
Blood Sugar			
Temperature			

Notes _____
_____
_____
_____

Date: _____ Wt. (am); _____ (pm); _____

Name: _____

	Morning	Mid-Day	Night
Blood Pressure	/	/	/
Heart Rate			
Oxygen Level			
Blood Sugar			
Temperature			

Notes _____
_____
_____
_____

Date:		Wt. (am);	(pm);
Name:			
	Morning	Mid-Day	Night
Blood Pressure	/	/	/
Heart Rate			
Oxygen Level			
Blood Sugar			
Temperature			

Notes _____
_____
_____
_____

Date:		Wt. (am);	(pm);
Name:			
	Morning	Mid-Day	Night
Blood Pressure	/	/	/
Heart Rate			
Oxygen Level			
Blood Sugar			
Temperature			

Notes _____
_____
_____
_____

Date:		Wt. (am);	(pm);
Name:			
	Morning	Mid-Day	Night
Blood Pressure	/	/	/
Heart Rate			
Oxygen Level			
Blood Sugar			
Temperature			

Notes _____
_____
_____
_____

Date:		Wt. (am);	(pm);
Name:			
	Morning	Mid-Day	Night
Blood Pressure	/	/	/
Heart Rate			
Oxygen Level			
Blood Sugar			
Temperature			

Notes _____
_____
_____
_____

Date:		Wt. (am);	(pm);
Name:			
	Morning	Mid-Day	Night
Blood Pressure	/	/	/
Heart Rate			
Oxygen Level			
Blood Sugar			
Temperature			

Notes _____

_____

_____

Date:		Wt. (am);	(pm);
Name:			
	Morning	Mid-Day	Night
Blood Pressure	/	/	/
Heart Rate			
Oxygen Level			
Blood Sugar			
Temperature			

Notes _____

_____

_____

Date:		Wt. (am);	(pm);
Name:			
	Morning	Mid-Day	Night
Blood Pressure	/	/	/
Heart Rate			
Oxygen Level			
Blood Sugar			
Temperature			

Notes _____
_____
_____
_____

Date:		Wt. (am);	(pm);
Name:			
	Morning	Mid-Day	Night
Blood Pressure	/	/	/
Heart Rate			
Oxygen Level			
Blood Sugar			
Temperature			

Notes _____
_____
_____
_____

Date:　　　　　　　　Wt. (am);　　　　　(pm);

Name:

	Morning	Mid-Day	Night
Blood Pressure	/	/	/
Heart Rate			
Oxygen Level			
Blood Sugar			
Temperature			

Notes _____

_____

_____

_____

Date:　　　　　　　　Wt. (am);　　　　　(pm);

Name:

	Morning	Mid-Day	Night
Blood Pressure	/	/	/
Heart Rate			
Oxygen Level			
Blood Sugar			
Temperature			

Notes _____

_____

_____

_____

Date:		Wt. (am);		(pm);
Name:				
	Morning	Mid-Day		Night
Blood Pressure	/	/		/
Heart Rate				
Oxygen Level				
Blood Sugar				
Temperature				

Notes _____
_____
_____
_____

Date:		Wt. (am);		(pm);
Name:				
	Morning	Mid-Day		Night
Blood Pressure	/	/		/
Heart Rate				
Oxygen Level				
Blood Sugar				
Temperature				

Notes _____
_____
_____
_____

Date:		Wt. (am);	(pm);
Name:			
	Morning	Mid-Day	Night
Blood Pressure	/	/	/
Heart Rate			
Oxygen Level			
Blood Sugar			
Temperature			

Notes _____

_____

_____

_____

Date:		Wt. (am);	(pm);
Name:			
	Morning	Mid-Day	Night
Blood Pressure	/	/	/
Heart Rate			
Oxygen Level			
Blood Sugar			
Temperature			

Notes _____

_____

_____

_____

Date:		Wt. (am);	(pm);
Name:			
	Morning	Mid-Day	Night
Blood Pressure	/	/	/
Heart Rate			
Oxygen Level			
Blood Sugar			
Temperature			

Notes _____
_____
_____
_____

Date:		Wt. (am);	(pm);
Name:			
	Morning	Mid-Day	Night
Blood Pressure	/	/	/
Heart Rate			
Oxygen Level			
Blood Sugar			
Temperature			

Notes _____
_____
_____
_____

Date:		Wt. (am);	(pm);
Name:			
	Morning	Mid-Day	Night
Blood Pressure	/	/	/
Heart Rate			
Oxygen Level			
Blood Sugar			
Temperature			

Notes _____
_____
_____
_____

Date:		Wt. (am);	(pm);
Name:			
	Morning	Mid-Day	Night
Blood Pressure	/	/	/
Heart Rate			
Oxygen Level			
Blood Sugar			
Temperature			

Notes _____
_____
_____
_____

Date:		Wt. (am);	(pm);
Name:			
	Morning	Mid-Day	Night
Blood Pressure	/	/	/
Heart Rate			
Oxygen Level			
Blood Sugar			
Temperature			

Notes _____
_____
_____
_____

Date:		Wt. (am);	(pm);
Name:			
	Morning	Mid-Day	Night
Blood Pressure	/	/	/
Heart Rate			
Oxygen Level			
Blood Sugar			
Temperature			

Notes _____
_____
_____
_____

Date:　　　　　　　　Wt. (am);　　　　　(pm);

Name:

	Morning	Mid-Day	Night
Blood Pressure	/	/	/
Heart Rate			
Oxygen Level			
Blood Sugar			
Temperature			

Notes _____
_____
_____
_____

Date:　　　　　　　　Wt. (am);　　　　　(pm);

Name:

	Morning	Mid-Day	Night
Blood Pressure	/	/	/
Heart Rate			
Oxygen Level			
Blood Sugar			
Temperature			

Notes _____
_____
_____
_____

Date:		Wt. (am);	(pm);
Name:			
	Morning	Mid-Day	Night
Blood Pressure	/	/	/
Heart Rate			
Oxygen Level			
Blood Sugar			
Temperature			

Notes _____
_____
_____
_____

Date:		Wt. (am);	(pm);
Name:			
	Morning	Mid-Day	Night
Blood Pressure	/	/	/
Heart Rate			
Oxygen Level			
Blood Sugar			
Temperature			

Notes _____
_____
_____
_____

Date:		Wt. (am);	(pm);
Name:			
	Morning	Mid-Day	Night
Blood Pressure	/	/	/
Heart Rate			
Oxygen Level			
Blood Sugar			
Temperature			

Notes _____
_____
_____
_____

Date:		Wt. (am);	(pm);
Name:			
	Morning	Mid-Day	Night
Blood Pressure	/	/	/
Heart Rate			
Oxygen Level			
Blood Sugar			
Temperature			

Notes _____
_____
_____
_____

Date:		Wt. (am);	(pm);
Name:			
	Morning	Mid-Day	Night
Blood Pressure	/	/	/
Heart Rate			
Oxygen Level			
Blood Sugar			
Temperature			

Notes _____
_____
_____
_____

Date:		Wt. (am);	(pm);
Name:			
	Morning	Mid-Day	Night
Blood Pressure	/	/	/
Heart Rate			
Oxygen Level			
Blood Sugar			
Temperature			

Notes _____
_____
_____
_____

Date:		Wt. (am);	(pm);
Name:			
	Morning	Mid-Day	Night
Blood Pressure	/	/	/
Heart Rate			
Oxygen Level			
Blood Sugar			
Temperature			

Notes _____
_____
_____
_____

Date:		Wt. (am);	(pm);
Name:			
	Morning	Mid-Day	Night
Blood Pressure	/	/	/
Heart Rate			
Oxygen Level			
Blood Sugar			
Temperature			

Notes _____
_____
_____
_____

Date:		Wt. (am);	(pm);
Name:			
	Morning	Mid-Day	Night
Blood Pressure	/	/	/
Heart Rate			
Oxygen Level			
Blood Sugar			
Temperature			

Notes _____
_____
_____
_____

Date:		Wt. (am);	(pm);
Name:			
	Morning	Mid-Day	Night
Blood Pressure	/	/	/
Heart Rate			
Oxygen Level			
Blood Sugar			
Temperature			

Notes _____
_____
_____
_____

Date: Wt. (am);   (pm);

Name:

	Morning	Mid-Day	Night
Blood Pressure	/	/	/
Heart Rate			
Oxygen Level			
Blood Sugar			
Temperature			

Notes _____
_____
_____
_____

Date: Wt. (am);   (pm);

Name:

	Morning	Mid-Day	Night
Blood Pressure	/	/	/
Heart Rate			
Oxygen Level			
Blood Sugar			
Temperature			

Notes _____
_____
_____
_____

Date:		Wt. (am);	(pm);
Name:			
	Morning	Mid-Day	Night
Blood Pressure	/	/	/
Heart Rate			
Oxygen Level			
Blood Sugar			
Temperature			

Notes _____
_____
_____
_____

Date:		Wt. (am);	(pm);
Name:			
	Morning	Mid-Day	Night
Blood Pressure	/	/	/
Heart Rate			
Oxygen Level			
Blood Sugar			
Temperature			

Notes _____
_____
_____
_____

Date:		Wt. (am);	(pm);
Name:			
	Morning	Mid-Day	Night
Blood Pressure	/	/	/
Heart Rate			
Oxygen Level			
Blood Sugar			
Temperature			

Notes _____

_____

_____

_____

Date:		Wt. (am);	(pm);
Name:			
	Morning	Mid-Day	Night
Blood Pressure	/	/	/
Heart Rate			
Oxygen Level			
Blood Sugar			
Temperature			

Notes _____

_____

_____

_____

Date:		Wt. (am);	(pm);
Name:			
	Morning	Mid-Day	Night
Blood Pressure	/	/	/
Heart Rate			
Oxygen Level			
Blood Sugar			
Temperature			

Notes _____
_____
_____
_____

Date:		Wt. (am);	(pm);
Name:			
	Morning	Mid-Day	Night
Blood Pressure	/	/	/
Heart Rate			
Oxygen Level			
Blood Sugar			
Temperature			

Notes _____
_____
_____
_____

Date: Wt. (am);   (pm);

Name:

	Morning	Mid-Day	Night
Blood Pressure	/	/	/
Heart Rate			
Oxygen Level			
Blood Sugar			
Temperature			

Notes _____

_____

_____

_____

Date: Wt. (am);   (pm);

Name:

	Morning	Mid-Day	Night
Blood Pressure	/	/	/
Heart Rate			
Oxygen Level			
Blood Sugar			
Temperature			

Notes _____

_____

_____

_____

Date:	Wt. (am);		(pm);
Name:			
	Morning	Mid-Day	Night
Blood Pressure	/	/	/
Heart Rate			
Oxygen Level			
Blood Sugar			
Temperature			

Notes _____
_____
_____

Date:	Wt. (am);		(pm);
Name:			
	Morning	Mid-Day	Night
Blood Pressure	/	/	/
Heart Rate			
Oxygen Level			
Blood Sugar			
Temperature			

Notes _____
_____
_____

Date: _____ Wt. (am); _____ (pm); _____

Name: _____

	Morning	Mid-Day	Night
Blood Pressure	/	/	/
Heart Rate			
Oxygen Level			
Blood Sugar			
Temperature			

Notes _____

_____

_____

Date: _____ Wt. (am); _____ (pm); _____

Name: _____

	Morning	Mid-Day	Night
Blood Pressure	/	/	/
Heart Rate			
Oxygen Level			
Blood Sugar			
Temperature			

Notes _____

_____

_____

Date:		Wt. (am);	(pm);
Name:			
	Morning	Mid-Day	Night
Blood Pressure	/	/	/
Heart Rate			
Oxygen Level			
Blood Sugar			
Temperature			

Notes _____
_____
_____
_____

Date:		Wt. (am);	(pm);
Name:			
	Morning	Mid-Day	Night
Blood Pressure	/	/	/
Heart Rate			
Oxygen Level			
Blood Sugar			
Temperature			

Notes _____
_____
_____
_____

Date:		Wt. (am);	(pm);
Name:			
	Morning	Mid-Day	Night
Blood Pressure	/	/	/
Heart Rate			
Oxygen Level			
Blood Sugar			
Temperature			

Notes _____

_____

_____

_____

Date:		Wt. (am);	(pm);
Name:			
	Morning	Mid-Day	Night
Blood Pressure	/	/	/
Heart Rate			
Oxygen Level			
Blood Sugar			
Temperature			

Notes _____

_____

_____

_____

Date:		Wt. (am);	(pm);
Name:			
	Morning	Mid-Day	Night
Blood Pressure	/	/	/
Heart Rate			
Oxygen Level			
Blood Sugar			
Temperature			

Notes _____
_____
_____
_____

Date:		Wt. (am);	(pm);
Name:			
	Morning	Mid-Day	Night
Blood Pressure	/	/	/
Heart Rate			
Oxygen Level			
Blood Sugar			
Temperature			

Notes _____
_____
_____
_____

Date: _____ Wt. (am); _____ (pm); _____

Name: _____

	Morning	Mid-Day	Night
Blood Pressure	/	/	/
Heart Rate			
Oxygen Level			
Blood Sugar			
Temperature			

Notes _____
_____
_____
_____

Date: _____ Wt. (am); _____ (pm); _____

Name: _____

	Morning	Mid-Day	Night
Blood Pressure	/	/	/
Heart Rate			
Oxygen Level			
Blood Sugar			
Temperature			

Notes _____
_____
_____
_____

Date:		Wt. (am);	(pm);
Name:			
	Morning	Mid-Day	Night
Blood Pressure	/	/	/
Heart Rate			
Oxygen Level			
Blood Sugar			
Temperature			

Notes _____
_____
_____
_____

Date:		Wt. (am);	(pm);
Name:			
	Morning	Mid-Day	Night
Blood Pressure	/	/	/
Heart Rate			
Oxygen Level			
Blood Sugar			
Temperature			

Notes _____
_____
_____
_____

Date:		Wt. (am);		(pm);
Name:				
	Morning	Mid-Day		Night
Blood Pressure	/	/		/
Heart Rate				
Oxygen Level				
Blood Sugar				
Temperature				

Notes _____

_____

_____

_____

Date:		Wt. (am);		(pm);
Name:				
	Morning	Mid-Day		Night
Blood Pressure	/	/		/
Heart Rate				
Oxygen Level				
Blood Sugar				
Temperature				

Notes _____

_____

_____

_____

Date: Wt. (am);   (pm);

Name:

	Morning	Mid-Day	Night
Blood Pressure	/	/	/
Heart Rate			
Oxygen Level			
Blood Sugar			
Temperature			

Notes _____
_____
_____
_____

Date: Wt. (am);   (pm);

Name:

	Morning	Mid-Day	Night
Blood Pressure	/	/	/
Heart Rate			
Oxygen Level			
Blood Sugar			
Temperature			

Notes _____
_____
_____
_____

Date:		Wt. (am);	(pm);
Name:			
	Morning	Mid-Day	Night
Blood Pressure	/	/	/
Heart Rate			
Oxygen Level			
Blood Sugar			
Temperature			

Notes _____
_____
_____
_____

Date:		Wt. (am);	(pm);
Name:			
	Morning	Mid-Day	Night
Blood Pressure	/	/	/
Heart Rate			
Oxygen Level			
Blood Sugar			
Temperature			

Notes _____
_____
_____
_____

Date:	Wt. (am);		(pm);
Name:			
	Morning	Mid-Day	Night
Blood Pressure	/	/	/
Heart Rate			
Oxygen Level			
Blood Sugar			
Temperature			

Notes _____
_____
_____

Date:	Wt. (am);		(pm);
Name:			
	Morning	Mid-Day	Night
Blood Pressure	/	/	/
Heart Rate			
Oxygen Level			
Blood Sugar			
Temperature			

Notes _____
_____
_____

Date: _____   Wt. (am); _____   (pm); _____

Name: _____

	Morning	Mid-Day	Night
Blood Pressure	/	/	/
Heart Rate			
Oxygen Level			
Blood Sugar			
Temperature			

Notes _____
_____
_____
_____

Date: _____   Wt. (am); _____   (pm); _____

Name: _____

	Morning	Mid-Day	Night
Blood Pressure	/	/	/
Heart Rate			
Oxygen Level			
Blood Sugar			
Temperature			

Notes _____
_____
_____
_____

Date:		Wt. (am);	(pm);
Name:			
	Morning	Mid-Day	Night
Blood Pressure	/	/	/
Heart Rate			
Oxygen Level			
Blood Sugar			
Temperature			

Notes _____
_____
_____
_____

Date:		Wt. (am);	(pm);
Name:			
	Morning	Mid-Day	Night
Blood Pressure	/	/	/
Heart Rate			
Oxygen Level			
Blood Sugar			
Temperature			

Notes _____
_____
_____
_____

Date:		Wt. (am);	(pm);
Name:			
	Morning	Mid-Day	Night
Blood Pressure	/	/	/
Heart Rate			
Oxygen Level			
Blood Sugar			
Temperature			

Notes _____

_____

_____

_____

Date:		Wt. (am);	(pm);
Name:			
	Morning	Mid-Day	Night
Blood Pressure	/	/	/
Heart Rate			
Oxygen Level			
Blood Sugar			
Temperature			

Notes _____

_____

_____

_____

Date:		Wt. (am);	(pm);
Name:			
	Morning	Mid-Day	Night
Blood Pressure	/	/	/
Heart Rate			
Oxygen Level			
Blood Sugar			
Temperature			

Notes _____
_____
_____
_____

Date:		Wt. (am);	(pm);
Name:			
	Morning	Mid-Day	Night
Blood Pressure	/	/	/
Heart Rate			
Oxygen Level			
Blood Sugar			
Temperature			

Notes _____
_____
_____
_____

Date: _____ Wt. (am); _____ (pm); _____

Name: _____

	Morning	Mid-Day	Night
Blood Pressure	/	/	/
Heart Rate			
Oxygen Level			
Blood Sugar			
Temperature			

Notes _____
_____
_____

Date: _____ Wt. (am); _____ (pm); _____

Name: _____

	Morning	Mid-Day	Night
Blood Pressure	/	/	/
Heart Rate			
Oxygen Level			
Blood Sugar			
Temperature			

Notes _____
_____
_____

Date:		Wt. (am);	(pm);
Name:			
	Morning	Mid-Day	Night
Blood Pressure	/	/	/
Heart Rate			
Oxygen Level			
Blood Sugar			
Temperature			

Notes _____
_____
_____
_____

Date:		Wt. (am);	(pm);
Name:			
	Morning	Mid-Day	Night
Blood Pressure	/	/	/
Heart Rate			
Oxygen Level			
Blood Sugar			
Temperature			

Notes _____
_____
_____
_____

Date:		Wt. (am);	(pm);
Name:			
	Morning	Mid-Day	Night
Blood Pressure	/	/	/
Heart Rate			
Oxygen Level			
Blood Sugar			
Temperature			

Notes _____
_____
_____
_____

Date:		Wt. (am);	(pm);
Name:			
	Morning	Mid-Day	Night
Blood Pressure	/	/	/
Heart Rate			
Oxygen Level			
Blood Sugar			
Temperature			

Notes _____
_____
_____
_____

Date:		Wt. (am);	(pm);
Name:			
	Morning	Mid-Day	Night
Blood Pressure	/	/	/
Heart Rate			
Oxygen Level			
Blood Sugar			
Temperature			

Notes _____
_____
_____
_____

Date:		Wt. (am);	(pm);
Name:			
	Morning	Mid-Day	Night
Blood Pressure	/	/	/
Heart Rate			
Oxygen Level			
Blood Sugar			
Temperature			

Notes _____
_____
_____
_____

Date: Wt. (am);   (pm);

Name:

	Morning	Mid-Day	Night
Blood Pressure	/	/	/
Heart Rate			
Oxygen Level			
Blood Sugar			
Temperature			

Notes _____

_____

_____

Date: Wt. (am);   (pm);

Name:

	Morning	Mid-Day	Night
Blood Pressure	/	/	/
Heart Rate			
Oxygen Level			
Blood Sugar			
Temperature			

Notes _____

_____

_____

Date:		Wt. (am);	(pm);
Name:			
	Morning	Mid-Day	Night
Blood Pressure	/	/	/
Heart Rate			
Oxygen Level			
Blood Sugar			
Temperature			

Notes _____
_____
_____
_____

Date:		Wt. (am);	(pm);
Name:			
	Morning	Mid-Day	Night
Blood Pressure	/	/	/
Heart Rate			
Oxygen Level			
Blood Sugar			
Temperature			

Notes _____
_____
_____
_____

Date:		Wt. (am);	(pm);
Name:			
	Morning	Mid-Day	Night
Blood Pressure	/	/	/
Heart Rate			
Oxygen Level			
Blood Sugar			
Temperature			

Notes _____

_____

_____

Date:		Wt. (am);	(pm);
Name:			
	Morning	Mid-Day	Night
Blood Pressure	/	/	/
Heart Rate			
Oxygen Level			
Blood Sugar			
Temperature			

Notes _____

_____

_____

Date:		Wt. (am);	(pm);
Name:			
	Morning	Mid-Day	Night
Blood Pressure	/	/	/
Heart Rate			
Oxygen Level			
Blood Sugar			
Temperature			

Notes _____
_____
_____
_____

Date:		Wt. (am);	(pm);
Name:			
	Morning	Mid-Day	Night
Blood Pressure	/	/	/
Heart Rate			
Oxygen Level			
Blood Sugar			
Temperature			

Notes _____
_____
_____
_____

Date:		Wt. (am);		(pm);
Name:				
	Morning	Mid-Day		Night
Blood Pressure	/	/		/
Heart Rate				
Oxygen Level				
Blood Sugar				
Temperature				

Notes _____

_____

_____

_____

Date:		Wt. (am);		(pm);
Name:				
	Morning	Mid-Day		Night
Blood Pressure	/	/		/
Heart Rate				
Oxygen Level				
Blood Sugar				
Temperature				

Notes _____

_____

_____

_____

Date:		Wt. (am);	(pm);
Name:			
	Morning	Mid-Day	Night
Blood Pressure	/	/	/
Heart Rate			
Oxygen Level			
Blood Sugar			
Temperature			

Notes _____
_____
_____
_____

Date:		Wt. (am);	(pm);
Name:			
	Morning	Mid-Day	Night
Blood Pressure	/	/	/
Heart Rate			
Oxygen Level			
Blood Sugar			
Temperature			

Notes _____
_____
_____
_____

Date:		Wt. (am);		(pm);
Name:				
	Morning	Mid-Day		Night
Blood Pressure	/	/		/
Heart Rate				
Oxygen Level				
Blood Sugar				
Temperature				

Notes _____

_____

_____

Date:		Wt. (am);		(pm);
Name:				
	Morning	Mid-Day		Night
Blood Pressure	/	/		/
Heart Rate				
Oxygen Level				
Blood Sugar				
Temperature				

Notes _____

_____

_____

Date:		Wt. (am);	(pm);
Name:			
	Morning	Mid-Day	Night
Blood Pressure	/	/	/
Heart Rate			
Oxygen Level			
Blood Sugar			
Temperature			

Notes _____
_____
_____
_____

Date:		Wt. (am);	(pm);
Name:			
	Morning	Mid-Day	Night
Blood Pressure	/	/	/
Heart Rate			
Oxygen Level			
Blood Sugar			
Temperature			

Notes _____
_____
_____
_____

Date:		Wt. (am);	(pm);
Name:			
	Morning	Mid-Day	Night
Blood Pressure	/	/	/
Heart Rate			
Oxygen Level			
Blood Sugar			
Temperature			

Notes _____
_____
_____
_____

Date:		Wt. (am);	(pm);
Name:			
	Morning	Mid-Day	Night
Blood Pressure	/	/	/
Heart Rate			
Oxygen Level			
Blood Sugar			
Temperature			

Notes _____
_____
_____
_____

Date:		Wt. (am);		(pm);	
Name:					
	Morning		Mid-Day		Night
Blood Pressure	/		/		/
Heart Rate					
Oxygen Level					
Blood Sugar					
Temperature					

Notes _____
_____
_____
_____

Date:		Wt. (am);		(pm);	
Name:					
	Morning		Mid-Day		Night
Blood Pressure	/		/		/
Heart Rate					
Oxygen Level					
Blood Sugar					
Temperature					

Notes _____
_____
_____
_____

Date: Wt. (am); (pm);

Name:

	Morning	Mid-Day	Night
Blood Pressure	/	/	/
Heart Rate			
Oxygen Level			
Blood Sugar			
Temperature			

Notes _____

_____

_____

_____

Date: Wt. (am); (pm);

Name:

	Morning	Mid-Day	Night
Blood Pressure	/	/	/
Heart Rate			
Oxygen Level			
Blood Sugar			
Temperature			

Notes _____

_____

_____

_____

Date:		Wt. (am);	(pm);
Name:			
	Morning	Mid-Day	Night
Blood Pressure	/	/	/
Heart Rate			
Oxygen Level			
Blood Sugar			
Temperature			

Notes _____
_____
_____
_____

Date:		Wt. (am);	(pm);
Name:			
	Morning	Mid-Day	Night
Blood Pressure	/	/	/
Heart Rate			
Oxygen Level			
Blood Sugar			
Temperature			

Notes _____
_____
_____
_____

Date:		Wt. (am);		(pm);	
Name:					
	Morning		Mid-Day		Night
Blood Pressure	/		/		/
Heart Rate					
Oxygen Level					
Blood Sugar					
Temperature					

Notes _____
_____
_____
_____

Date:		Wt. (am);		(pm);	
Name:					
	Morning		Mid-Day		Night
Blood Pressure	/		/		/
Heart Rate					
Oxygen Level					
Blood Sugar					
Temperature					

Notes _____
_____
_____
_____

Date:		Wt. (am);	(pm);
Name:			
	Morning	Mid-Day	Night
Blood Pressure	/	/	/
Heart Rate			
Oxygen Level			
Blood Sugar			
Temperature			

Notes _____
_____
_____

Date:		Wt. (am);	(pm);
Name:			
	Morning	Mid-Day	Night
Blood Pressure	/	/	/
Heart Rate			
Oxygen Level			
Blood Sugar			
Temperature			

Notes _____
_____
_____

Date: Wt. (am);   (pm);

Name:

	Morning	Mid-Day	Night
Blood Pressure	/	/	/
Heart Rate			
Oxygen Level			
Blood Sugar			
Temperature			

Notes _____

_____

_____

_____

Date: Wt. (am);   (pm);

Name:

	Morning	Mid-Day	Night
Blood Pressure	/	/	/
Heart Rate			
Oxygen Level			
Blood Sugar			
Temperature			

Notes _____

_____

_____

_____

Date:		Wt. (am);	(pm);
Name:			
	Morning	Mid-Day	Night
Blood Pressure	/	/	/
Heart Rate			
Oxygen Level			
Blood Sugar			
Temperature			

Notes _____
_____
_____
_____

Date:		Wt. (am);	(pm);
Name:			
	Morning	Mid-Day	Night
Blood Pressure	/	/	/
Heart Rate			
Oxygen Level			
Blood Sugar			
Temperature			

Notes _____
_____
_____
_____

Date: Wt. (am);   (pm);

Name:

	Morning	Mid-Day	Night
Blood Pressure	/	/	/
Heart Rate			
Oxygen Level			
Blood Sugar			
Temperature			

Notes _____

_____

_____

_____

Date: Wt. (am);   (pm);

Name:

	Morning	Mid-Day	Night
Blood Pressure	/	/	/
Heart Rate			
Oxygen Level			
Blood Sugar			
Temperature			

Notes _____

_____

_____

_____

Date:		Wt. (am);	(pm);
Name:			
	Morning	Mid-Day	Night
Blood Pressure	/	/	/
Heart Rate			
Oxygen Level			
Blood Sugar			
Temperature			

Notes _____
_____
_____
_____

Date:		Wt. (am);	(pm);
Name:			
	Morning	Mid-Day	Night
Blood Pressure	/	/	/
Heart Rate			
Oxygen Level			
Blood Sugar			
Temperature			

Notes _____
_____
_____
_____

Date:		Wt. (am);		(pm);
Name:				
	Morning	Mid-Day		Night
Blood Pressure	/	/		/
Heart Rate				
Oxygen Level				
Blood Sugar				
Temperature				

Notes _____

_____

_____

Date:		Wt. (am);		(pm);
Name:				
	Morning	Mid-Day		Night
Blood Pressure	/	/		/
Heart Rate				
Oxygen Level				
Blood Sugar				
Temperature				

Notes _____

_____

_____

Date:		Wt. (am);	(pm);
Name:			
	Morning	Mid-Day	Night
Blood Pressure	/	/	/
Heart Rate			
Oxygen Level			
Blood Sugar			
Temperature			

Notes _____
_____
_____
_____

Date:		Wt. (am);	(pm);
Name:			
	Morning	Mid-Day	Night
Blood Pressure	/	/	/
Heart Rate			
Oxygen Level			
Blood Sugar			
Temperature			

Notes _____
_____
_____
_____

Thank You For Shopping With us

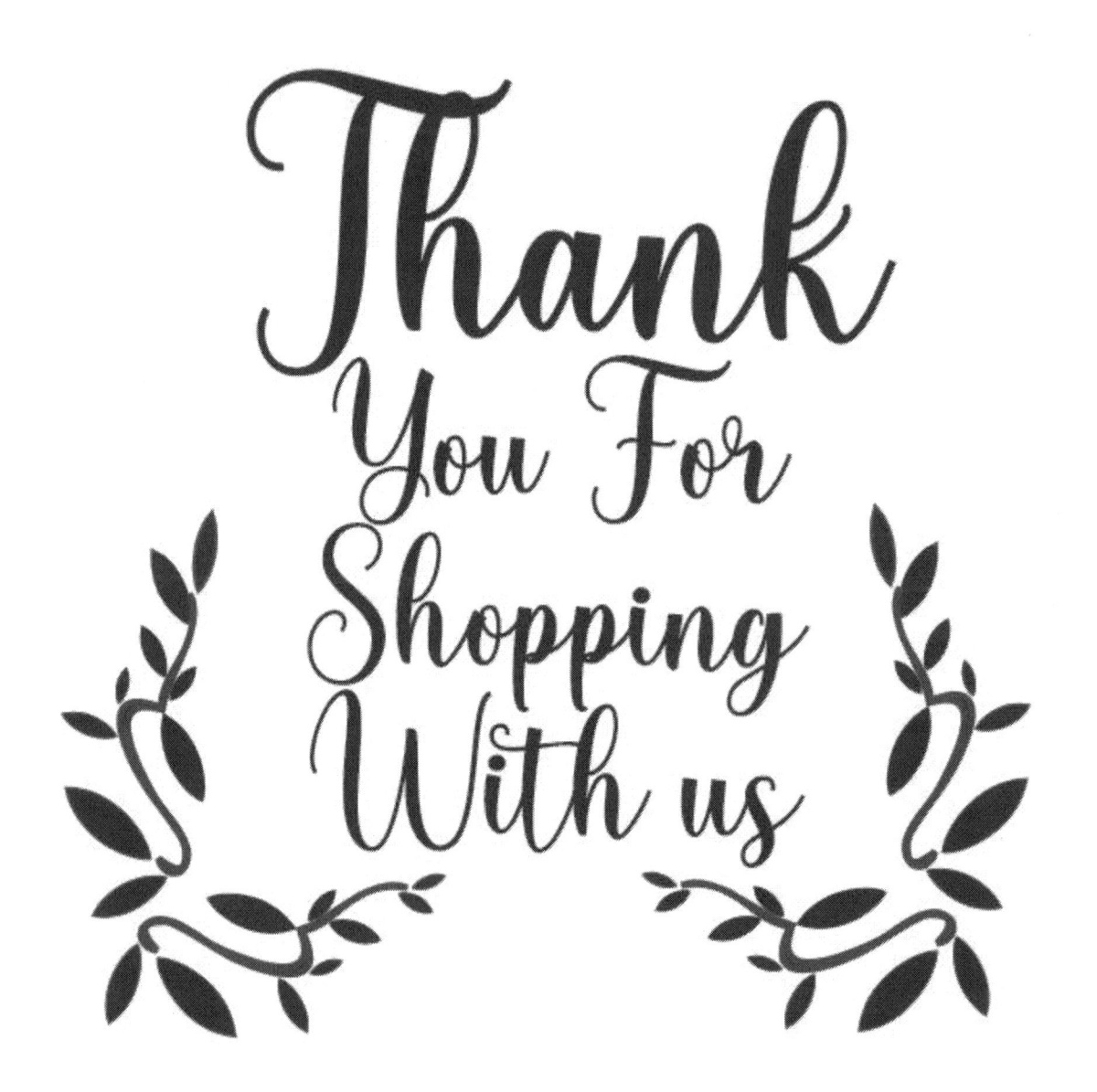

Copyright © All Rights Reserved by Logbooks Simon

Made in the USA
Columbia, SC
09 January 2025